Inter

Fasting Recipes Collection

The Complete Step-by-Step Guide to Lose Weight, Reset Metabolism and Stay Fit with Tasty Recipes.

Tim Farrell

Additionally, the information in the following pages is intended only for informational purposes and should thus be thought of as universal. As befitting its nature, it is presented without assurance regarding its prolonged validity or interim quality. Trademarks that are mentioned are done without written consent and can in no way be considered an endorsement from the trademark holder.

Table of Contents

BREAKFAST

1. Delicious Flax Pancakes

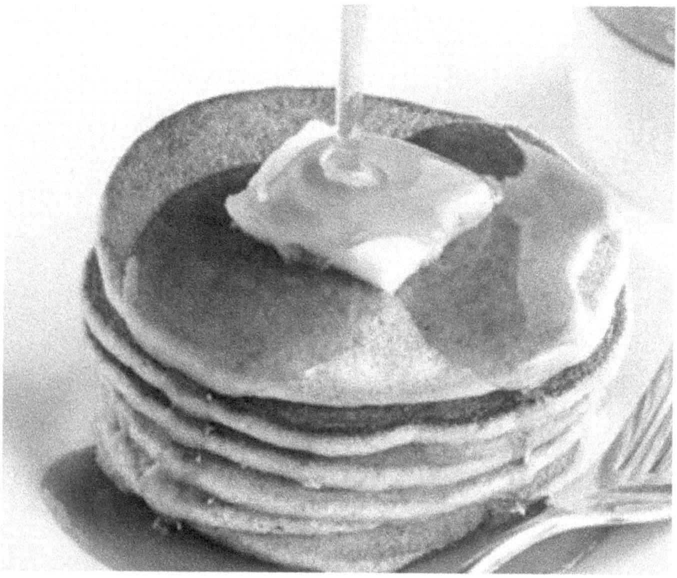

Preparation Time: 5 minutes

Cooking Time: 20 minutes

Servings: 3

Ingredients:

- 150 g of fat sour cream
- 4 eggs
- ½ tsp. of salt
- 1 tsp. of baking powder
- 50 g of room temperature butter
- 6 tsp. with a hill of ground flax seeds
- sweetener to taste
- 20 g of any fat for frying

Directions:

1. Using a mixer, beat the butter, add the eggs, sour cream, baking powder, salt, and sweetener and beat until smooth all together
2. Add one spoonful of flax and continue to whisk.
3. The dough should turn out as it is for pancakes, that is, as a thick sour cream.
4. Heat the pan, put the oil in and fry as usual. But layout the circles thickly and with a diameter of about 4 cm, because they sprawl out and become larger.
5. Fry over low heat, otherwise they will burn.

Nutrition: Carbohydrates: 1.42 g Fats: 7.20 g Proteins: 2.08 g Calories: 75.69

2. Homemade Bacon and Egg Burgers

Preparation Time: 10 minutes

Cooking Time: 30 minutes

Servings: 3

Ingredients:

- 6 eggs
- 3 tbsp. of nutmeg, I used peanut
- 50 g of butter, melted
- salt, black pepper to taste
- Ingredients for the filling
- 9 strips of bacon
- 3 eggs

Directions:

1. Mix the ingredients for the pancakes and fry as usual. To make them perfectly round, it is better to use silicone molds for pancakes or scrambled eggs.
2. Fry three eggs. It is advisable to use forms too.
3. Fry the bacon.

4. Combine all the ingredients in the form of a burger, in addition, use everything you want: herbs, cucumbers, cheese or salsa sauce.

Nutrition: Carbohydrates: 3.2 g Fats: 35.8 g Proteins: 26.78 g Calories: 447.62

3. Almond Flour Pancakes

Preparation Time: 5 minutes

Cooking Time: 5 minutes

Servings: 4

Ingredients

- ½ cup almond flour
- ½ cup cream cheese
- 4 medium eggs
- ½ tsp cinnamon
- ½ tsp granulated sweetener
- 1 tsp grass-fed butter
- 1 tbsp sugar-free syrup

Directions

1. Add all the ingredients into a blender and let them blend in well. Once done, set the batter aside.
2. On a non-stick pan at medium heat, fry pancakes with melted butter. Once the center starts to bubble, turn over. Once done with the pancake, move on to the rest, using the batter.
3. Finally, serve your pancakes warm, along with some low carb fruit or with an exquisite side of

sugar-free syrup to enjoy a healthy and tasty breakfast.

Nutrition: Calories: 234 Fat: 20g Carbohydrates: 4g Fiber: 1.5g Net carbs: 2.5g Protein: 11g

4. Avocado Toast

Preparation Time: 20 minutes

Cooking Time: 40 minutes

Servings: 2

Ingredients

- ½ cup grass-fed butter
- 2 tbsp coconut oil
- 7 large eggs
- 1 tsp baking powder
- 2 cups almond flour
- ½ tsp xanthan gum
- ½ tsp kosher salt
- 1 medium avocado

Directions

1. Preheat over at 3500F. Beat eggs for around two minutes with a mixer at high speed. Then, add coconut oil and butter (both melted) to the eggs and continue beating. Ensure that oil and butter are not too warm to cook the eggs. Add remaining bread ingredients and mix well. Now, the batter should become thick. Pour batter in a non-stick

loaf pan lined with parchment paper. Let it bake for 45 minutes or until the fork comes clean through the middle.

2. For topping, toast two slices of your intermittent bread to your liking. Slice the whole avocado thinly, without the skin or pit. Use these to make one long strip of overlapping slices. Roll these into a spiral and that is it! Enjoy your intermittent bread with avocado topping.

Nutrition: Calories: 350 Fat: 32g Carbohydrates: 7g Fiber: 4g Net carbs: 3g Protein: 10g

5. Chicken Avocado Egg Bacon Salad

Preparation Time: 10 minutes

Cooking Time: 10 minutes

Servings: 4

Ingredients

- 12 oz. cooked chicken breast
- 6 slices crumbled bacon
- 3 boiled eggs cut into cubes
- 1 cup cherry tomatoes cut into halves
- 1/2 small sliced red onion
- 1 large avocado(s)
- 1/2 stick finely chopped celery
- Salad Dressing
- 1/2 cup olive oil mayonnaise
- 2 tbsp. sour cream
- 1 tsp Dijon mustard
- 4 tbsp. extra virgin olive oil
- 2 cloves minced garlic
- 2 tsp lemon juice
- 4 cups lettuce

- Salt and pepper to taste

Directions

1. Combine all the ingredients together and mix them well for the salad dressing. Then, combine chicken, tomatoes, bacon, eggs, red onions, and celery together. Add about ¾ of the salad dressing and mix them well. Add the avocado and toss together gently. Check the taste and, if needed, add the remainder of the salad dressing as well. Finally, add salt and pepper to taste and then serve it over lettuce.

Nutrition: Calories: 387 Fat: 27g Carbohydrates: 2.5g Fiber: 1g Net carbs: 1.5g Protein: 24g

6. Bacon Wrapped Chicken Breast

Preparation Time: 10 minutes

Cooking Time: 45 minutes

Servings: 4

Ingredients

- 4 boneless, skinless chicken breast
- 8 oz. sharp cheddar cheese
- 8 slices bacon
- 4 oz. sliced jalapeno peppers
- 1 tsp garlic powder
- Salt and pepper to taste

Directions

1. Preheat the oven at around 3500F. Ensure to season both sides of chicken breast well with salt, garlic powder, and pepper. Place the chicken breast on a non-stick baking sheet (foil-covered). Cover the chicken with cheese and add jalapeno slices. Cut the bacon slices in half and then place the four halves over each piece of chicken. Bake for around 30 to 45 minutes at most. If the chicken is set but the bacon still feels

undercooked, you may want to put it under the broiler for a few minutes. Once done, serve hot with a side of low carb garlic parmesan roasted asparagus.

Nutrition: Calories: 640 Fat: 48g Carbohydrates: 6g Fiber: 3g Net carbs: 3g Protein: 47g

7. Egg Salad

Preparation Time: 15 minutes

Cooking Time: 10 minutes

Servings: 4

Ingredients

- 6 eggs
- 2 tbsp mayonnaise
- 1 tsp Dijon mustard
- 1 tsp lemon juice
- Salt and pepper to taste

Directions

1. In a medium saucepan, place the solid eggs gently.
2. Add some cold water so that the eggs are covered around an inch. Boil them for around 10 minutes.
3. Once done, remove them from the heat and let them cool. Peel the eggs while running them under cold water. Now add these in a food processor and pulse until they are chopped.

4. Add and stir mayonnaise, lemon juice, mustard, and salt and pepper. Ensure to taste and then adjust as necessary.
5. Finally, serve them with a bit of lettuce leaves and, if needed, bacon for wrapping.

Nutrition: Calories: 222 Fat: 19g Net carbs: 1g Protein: 13g

8. Blueberry Muffins

Preparation Time: 10 minutes

Cooking Time: 30 minutes

Servings: 12

Ingredients

- 1 container Greek yogurt
- 3 large eggs
- 1/2 tsp vanilla extract
- 1/4 tsp salt
- 2 1/2 cups almond flour
- 1/4 cup Swerve sweetener (add more if using plain Greek yogurt)
- 2 tsp baking powder
- Water if needed to thin
- 1/2 cup fresh blueberries

Directions

1. Preheat oven at 325°F. Simultaneously, line-up a clean muffin pan with around 12 parchment liners. Combine yogurt, vanilla, eggs, and salt in a blender. Blend the mixture till it is smooth. Add almond flour, baking powder and sweetener.

Now, blend again until it is smooth. If the batter is thick, add one tablespoon of water at a time. The batter should be thick, but it must be pourable.

2. Add in blueberries and divide these equally for the prepared muffin cups. Finally, bake these for 25 to 30 minutes. Use a tester and insert it right in the middle. If it comes out clean, your muffins are ready.

Nutrition: Calories: 163 Net carbs: 3.8g Fat: 12.9g Protein: 7.6g

LUNCH

9. Chicken Pizzaiola

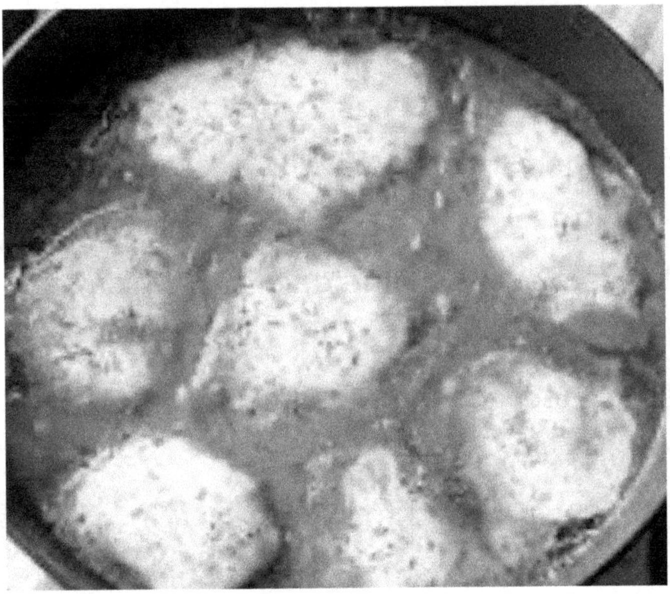

Preparation Time: 10 minutes

Cooking Time: 20 minutes

Servings: 3

Ingredients:

- 3 chicken breasts
- 1 tray with ham

- 1 cup pasta sauce
- 1 and ½ cups grated cheese
- 1 Pinch of salt and pepper
- 2 Tbsps. olive oil

Directions:

1. Preheat the oven to 290 °F
2. Place the 3 chicken breasts on a sheet of parchment paper directly on the plate of your oven.
3. Slice the breasts partially and garnish with sauce, ham, and cheese.
4. Cover with grated cheese, season with salt and pepper and drizzle with oil.
5. Bake in a hot oven for 20 minutes
6. Once ready, divide the 2 chicken breasts between three containers
7. Seal the containers very well and store it in the refrigerator for 3 days

Nutrition: Calories: 453 Fat: 34.8 g Carbs: 8.9 g Protein 26g Sugar: 1.5 g

10. Beef Stroganoff with Protein Noodles

Preparation Time: 14 minutes

Cooking Time: 29 min

Servings: 1

Ingredients:

- 2 oz. Barilla Protein Farfalle Pasta
- ½ cup fresh sliced mushrooms
- 2 Tbsp of chopped onion
- 1 T butter
- dash of black pepper
- 6 oz. steak, sliced thinly
- 1 T tomato paste
- ¼ tsp of Dijon mustard
- ½ cup beef broth
- ½ small container plain Greek yogurt

Directions:

1. Cook the pasta in water.
2. Place the butter in a Teflon skillet.
3. Next add in the onions, and mushrooms, cook until onions are shiny and water is gone.

4. Add the beef and brown well.
5. Stir in remaining ingredients except the pasta and yogurt.
6. Cook this until the beef is done, approximately 9 minutes.
7. Drain the pasta.
8. If the sauce is too thin, add 1 tsp low carb flax meal and boil to thicken.
9. Turn back down to low. Then add the yogurt to the sauce.
10. Serve the stroganoff over the pasta.

Nutrition: Calories: 559 Total Fat: 23g; Protein: 55gTotal Carbs: 4g Dietary Fiber: 13gSugar: 2gSodium: 957mg

11. Beefy Tostadas

Preparation Time: 4 minute

Cooking Time: 9 minutes

Servings: 2

Ingredients:

- ¼ pound ground sirloin
- ¼ cup onions, minced
- 1 tsp garlic, minced
- 1 T olive oil
- ½ cup chopped green, red, and yellow peppers
- ½ cup cheddar cheese, mild or sharp, hand-shredded
- 2 Tortilla factory low-carb tortillas
- 2 T butter
- 1 c Greek yogurt, plain
- 2 T salsa Verde

Directions:

1. Brown the tortillas in the butter. Place on a warm plate.
2. Cook the sirloin, onions, garlic, peppers in the olive oil.

3. Place on the tortillas.
4. Top with the cheese.
5. Add the Greek yogurt.
6. Drizzle with the salsa.

Nutrition: Calories: 735 Total Fat: 48g Protein: 66g Total Carbs: 18g Dietary Fiber: 8g Sugar: 0g Sodium: 708mg

12. Bratwurst German Dinner

Preparation Time: 4 minutes

Cooking Time: 19 minutes

Servings:

Ingredients:

- 1 Bratwurst sausage
- ½ cup sliced onion
- ½ cup sauerkraut, this includes the liquid
- 1 tsp olive oil
- Sprinkle of black pepper

Directions:

1. Cook the bratwurst and the onion in the olive oil, in a coated skillet.
2. Remove the bratwurst to a plate.
3. Place the sauerkraut into the skillet and cook 3 min.
4. Add the bratwurst and onion back to warm and mingle the flavors.
5. Sprinkle with black pepper and serve.

Nutrition: Calories: 332 Total Fat: 26g Protein: 15g Total Carbs: 8g Dietary Fiber: 9g Sugar: 4g Sodium: 1188mg

13. Cajun Blackened Fish with Cauliflower Salad

Preparation Time: 9 minutes

Cooking Time: 9 minutes

Servings: 1

Ingredients:

- 1 cup chopped cauliflower
- 1 tsp red pepper flakes
- 1 T Italian seasonings
- 1 T garlic, minced
- 6 oz. tilapia
- 1 cup English cucumber, chopped with peel
- 2 T olive oil
- 1 sprig dill, chopped
- 1 Sweetener packet
- 3 T lime juice
- 2 T Cajun blackened seasoning

Directions:

1. Mix the seasonings, except the Cajun blackened seasoning, into one bowl.
2. Add 1 T olive oil.

3. Emulsify or whip.
4. Pour the dressing over the cauliflower and cucumber.
5. Brush the fish with the olive oil on both sides.
6. Pour the other 1 T oil into a coated skillet.
7. Press the Cajun seasoning onto both sides of the fish.
8. Cook the fish in the olive oil 3 minutes per side.
9. Plate and serve.

Nutrition: Calories: 530 Total Fat: 33.5g Protein: 32g Total Carbs: 5.5g Dietary Fiber: 4g Sugar: 3g Sodium: 80mg

14. Chicken Parmesan over Protein Pasta

Preparation Time: 9 minutes

Cooking Time: 14 minutes

Servings: 2

Ingredients:

- 1 dash black pepper
- ½ tsp Italian spice mix
- 8 oz. Protein Plus Spaghetti
- ½ hand-shredded Parmesan
- 1 diced zucchini squash
- 1 ½ cups marinara sauce, any brand
- 24 oz. boneless thin chicken cutlets
- 2 T olive oil
- ½ cup grated Mozzarella cheese
- Water, for boiling the pasta

Directions:

1. Boil the pasta with the zucchini in the water.
2. Mix the Italian spices and ¼ cup Parmesan cheese and place in a shallow dish.

3. Brush the chicken pieces with olive oil and press into spice and cheese to coat.
4. Place in skillet with the oil and cook until done.
5. Add the marinara sauce to the skillet to warm, cover the chicken if you desire.
6. Drain the pasta and zucchini, place on plates.
7. Top the chicken with the mozzarella and remaining Parmesan cheese.
8. Place sauce, chicken, and cheese onto spaghetti and serve.

Nutrition: Calories: 372 Total Fat: 18g Protein: 56g Total Carbs: 7 g Dietary Fiber: 2g Sugar: 6g Sodium: 1335mg

15. Chicken Chow Mein Stir Fry

Preparation Time: 9 minutes

Cooking Time: 14 minutes

Servings: 4

Ingredients:

- 1/2 cup sliced onion
- 2 T Oil, sesame garlic flavored
- 4 cups shredded Bok-Choy
- 1 c Sugar Snap Peas
- 1 cup fresh bean sprouts
- 3 stalks Celery, chopped
- 1 1/2 tsp minced Garlic
- 1 packet Splenda
- 1 cup Broth, chicken
- 2 T Soy Sauce
- 1 T ginger, freshly minced
- 1 tsp cornstarch
- 4 boneless Chicken Breasts, cooked/sliced thinly

Directions:

1. Place the bok-choy, peas, celery in a skillet with 1 T garlic oil.

2. Stir fry until bok-choy is softened to liking.
3. Add remaining ingredients except the cornstarch.
4. If too thin, stir cornstarch into ½ cup cold water. When smooth pour into skillet.
5. Bring cornstarch and chow mein to a one-minute boil. Turn off the heat source.
6. Stir sauce then for wait 4 minutes to serve, after the chow mein has thickened.

Nutrition: Calories: 368 Total Fat: 18g Protein: 42g Total Carbs: 12g Dietary Fiber: 16g Sugar: 6g Sodium: 746mg

DINNER

16. Slow-Cooked Salsa Chicken

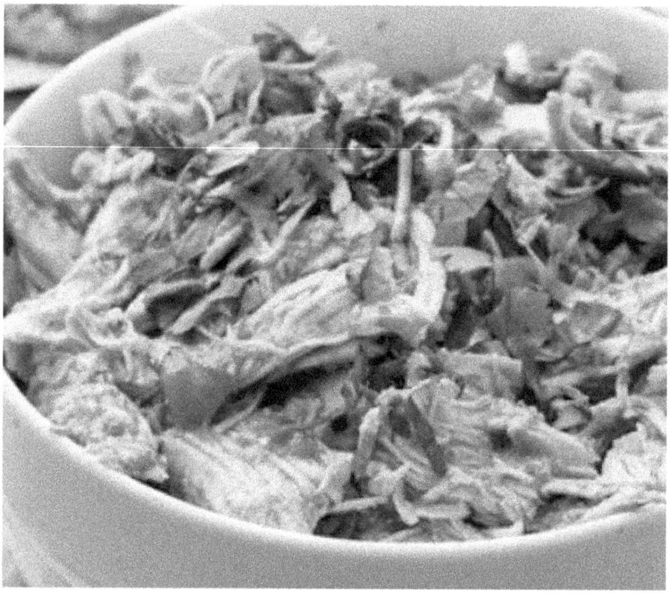

Preparation Time: 5 minutes

Cooking Time: 2 hours

Servings: 6

Ingredients:

- 3 pounds of boneless, skinless chicken breasts
- 2 cups of mild salsa

- 1 cup of shredded Mexican Blend cheese

Direction

1. Place the chicken to your slow cooker and add the mild salsa.
2. Cover with a lid. Cook on "High" for 1 hour and 30 minutes to 2 hours.
3. Preheat your oven to 425 degrees Fahrenheit.
4. Transfer the chicken to a greased baking dish and sprinkle with the Mexican blend cheese.
5. Place inside your oven and bake for 15 minutes or until golden brown.
6. Serve and enjoy!

Nutrition: calories 351, fat 9g, fiber 1g, carbs 8g, protein 54g

17. Chicken with Mustard Sauce and Bacon

Preparation Time: 10 minutes

Cooking Time: 30 minutes

Servings: 3

Ingredients:

- 2 pounds of boneless, skinless chicken breast
- 1/3 cup of Dijon mustard
- ¼ teaspoon of fine sea salt
- ¼ teaspoon of smoked paprika or regular paprika
- 8 medium bacon slices, finely chopped
- 1 small white or red onion, finely chopped
- 1 tablespoon of extra-virgin olive oil
- 1 ½ cups of homemade low-sodium chicken broth

Direction

1. In a small bowl, add the Dijon mustard, smoked paprika, fine sea salt, and freshly cracked black pepper. Stir until well combined.
2. Baste the Dijon mustard mixture all over the chicken breast.

3. In a large skillet over medium-high heat, add the bacon and cook until brown and crispy. Transfer to a plate lined with paper towels.
4. Add 1 tablespoon of extra-virgin olive oil to the skillet. Add the chicken and cook for 2 minutes per side. Transfer the chicken to a plate.
5. Pour in the chicken broth to the skillet and raise the heat until begins to bubble. Return the cooked bacon and chopped onions to the skillet.
6. Return the chicken to the skillet and reduce the heat. Cover with a lid and allow to simmer for 15 to 20 minutes or until the chicken is thoroughly cooked.
7. Serve and enjoy!

Nutrition: calories 681, fat 9g, fiber 2g, carbs 8g, protein 74g

18. Incredibly Delicious Lasagna

Preparation Time: 10 minutes

Cooking Time: 1 hour 30 minutes

Servings: 4

Ingredients:

- 1 pound of lean grass-fed ground beef
- 1 (16-ounce) package of lasagna noodles
- 1 cup of shredded mozzarella cheese
- 1 onion, finely chopped
- ½ cup of mushrooms, finely chopped
- 1 pint of ricotta cheese
- ¼ cup of parmesan cheese, finely grated
- 2 eggs
- 1 (28-ounce) jar of spaghetti sauce
- 1 (16-ounce) package of cottage cheese

Direction

1. Preheat your oven to 350 degrees Fahrenheit.
2. In a large skillet over medium-high heat, add the ground beef and cook until brown.

3. Add the chopped mushrooms and onions. Cook until the mushrooms and onions have softened, stirring occasionally.
4. Stir in the spaghetti sauce and allow to heat through.
5. In a medium bowl, add the cottage cheese, ricotta cheese, and parmesan grated cheese, and eggs. Stir until well combined.
6. Spread a layer of the meat mixture to a greased baking dish.
7. Layer with lasagna noodles.
8. Spread the cheese mixture over the lasagna noodles and sprinkle with the mozzarella cheese.
9. Add another layer of meat mixture and repeat with all the ingredients. Make sure you have ½ cup of shredded mozzarella cheese left.
10. Cover the baking dish with foil and place inside your oven. Bake for 45 minutes.
11. Remove the aluminum foil and sprinkle with the remaining ½ cup of shredded mozzarella cheese. Bake for 15 minutes.
12. Remove from your oven and allow to cool. Serve and enjoy!

Nutrition: calories 712, fat 31g, fiber 6g, carbs 50g, protein 44g

19. Beef Stroganoff

Preparation Time: 10 minutes

Cooking Time: 30 minutes

Servings: 6

Ingredients:

- 1(10-ounce) package of egg noodles, cooked according to the package Direction
- 2 pounds of beef steak, sliced into thin strips
- 4 tablespoons of butter
- 2 cups of brown or cremini mushrooms, sliced
- 1 large white or yellow onion, sliced
- 2 medium garlic cloves, minced
- ½ cup of sour cream
- ¼ cup of flour
- 2 teaspoons of Worcestershire sauce
- 1 teaspoon of Dijon mustard
- 1 teaspoon of smoked paprika or regular paprika
- 3 cups of homemade low-sodium beef stock
- ½ teaspoon of fine sea salt
- ½ teaspoon of freshly cracked black pepper

Direction

1. In a large skillet over medium-high heat, add 2 tablespoons of butter.
2. Add the beef strips and cook until brown. Remove and set aside.
3. Add the remaining 2 tablespoons of butter to the skillet along with the sliced mushrooms, chopped onion and minced garlic. Sauté until vegetables have softened, stirring occasionally.
4. Sprinkle ¼ cup of flour over the vegetables and cook for another minute, stirring occasionally.
5. Lower the heat and stir in the beef stock while whisking constantly. Allow to simmer until thickens.
6. Stir in the Worcestershire sauce, Dijon mustard, smoked paprika and sour cream until well combined.
7. Stir in the beef strips and simmer for another 5 minutes.
8. Serve over egg noodles.

Nutrition: calories 497, fat 22g, fiber 2g, carbs 19g, protein 49g

20. Tasteful Beef Burrito Skillet

Preparation Time: 10 minutes

Cooking Time: 20 minutes

Servings: 6

Ingredients:

- 1 pound of lean grass-fed ground beef
- 1 (1-ounce) package of taco seasoning mix
- 1 cup of mild chunky salsa
- 4 flour tortillas, sliced into strips
- 1 (15-ounce) can of black beans, drained and rinsed
- 1 cup of water
- 1 cup of shredded Mexican blend cheese
- ½ cup of sour cream
- ¼ cup of green onions, sliced

Direction

1. In a large nonstick skillet over medium-high heat, add the ground beef. Cook until brown, stirring occasionally. Drain the excess liquid.
2. Add the taco seasoning mix, mild chunky salsa and black beans. Reduce the heat.

3. Stir in the tortilla strips and top with the shredded Mexican blend cheese. Remove from the heat and allow the cheese to melt.
4. Top with sour cream and sprinkle with sliced green onions
5. Serve and enjoy!

Nutrition: calories 384, fat 21g, fiber 7g, carbs 28g, protein 24g

21. Freekeh Salad

Preparation Time: 10 minutes

Cooking Time: 10 minutes

Servings: 2

Ingredients:

- 2 vine tomatoes, chopped or 4 cherry tomatoes, quartered
- Sea salt to taste
- 2 tbsp olive oil
- Juice of ½ lemon
- Zest of ½ lemon, grated
- A handful fresh cilantro or parsley, chopped
- 1 small cucumber, chopped
- ½ cup corn kernels
- 1 small onion, chopped
- ¾ cup freekeh
- 2 cups water

To serve:

- Hummus or pesto as required
- Avocado slices
- Mini tortillas or wraps, as required

Direction:

1. Add freekeh and water. Place water over medium heat. When it begins to boil, lower the heat and cover with a lid. Simmer for 10-12 minutes. Uncover and cook until tender. Drain and set aside.
2. Add lemon juice, oil, zest, salt and pepper into a small bowl and whisk well.
3. Add rest of the ingredients including freekeh into a bowl and toss well. Pour dressing on top and toss well. Chill until ready to use.
4. Spread tortillas on your countertop. Place salad on one half of the tortillas. Top with avocado and hummus. Fold the other half over the filling and serve.

Nutrition: calories 800, fat 8g, fiber 2g, carbs 12g, protein 69g

22. Kamut, Lentil, and Chickpea Soup

Preparation Time: 10 minutes

Cooking Time: 50 minutes

Servings: 9

Ingredients:

- ½ cups kamut berries, rinsed
- 4 tbsp olive oil
- 2 cups carrots, finely chopped
- 1 cup celery, thinly sliced
- 4 tsp fresh thyme, chopped
- 4 cloves garlic, minced
- 4 bay leaves
- ½ tsp pepper powder
- A handful celery leaves, chopped (optional)
- 4 cups boiling water
- 4 cups onion, finely chopped
- 1 ½ cups fresh parsley, chopped
- 2 tbsp chopped fresh thyme
- 8 cans (14.5 ounces each) chicken broth or use equivalent homemade broth

- 2/3 cup dried lentils, rinsed, soaked in water for 20 minutes
- 2 cans (15 ounces each) chickpeas, rinsed, drained

Direction:

1. Add kamut into a bowl. Cover with boiling water. Let it soak for 30 minutes.
2. Place a soup pot over medium heat. Add oil. When the oil is heated, add onion and herbs and sauté until onions are translucent.
3. Add garlic and saute until fragrant.
4. Add rest of the ingredients except chickpeas and stir. Cover and cook until tender.
5. Ladle into soup bowls. Sprinkle celery and serve.

Nutrition: calories 800, fat 8g, fiber 2g, carbs 12g, protein 69g

23. Cheesy Garlic Bread with Smoked Salmon

Preparation Time: 10 minutes

Cooking Time: 1 minute;

Servings: 2

Ingredients

- 4 tbsp. almond flour
- ½ tsp baking powder
- 2 tbsp. grated cheddar cheese
- 1 egg
- 2 oz. salmon, cut into thin sliced
- Seasoning:
- 1 tbsp. butter, unsalted
- ¼ tsp garlic powder
- 1/8 tsp salt
- ¼ tsp Italian seasoning

Directions:

1. Take a heatproof bowl, place all the ingredients in it except for cheese and then stir by using a fork until well combined.

2. Fold in cheese until just mixed and then microwave for 1 minute at high heat setting until thoroughly cooked, else continue cooking for another 15 to 30 seconds.
3. When done, lift out the bread, cool it for 5 minutes and then cut it into slices.
4. Top each slice with salmon and then serve straight away

Nutrition: 233 Calories; 18 g Fats; 13.8 g Protein; 1.9 g Net Carb; 1.5 g Fiber;

24. Smoked Salmon Pasta Salad

Preparation Time: 10 minutes

Cooking Time: 0 minutes;

Servings: 2

Ingredients

- 1 zucchini, spiralized into noodles
- 4 oz. smoked salmon, break into pieces
- 2 oz. cream cheese
- 2 oz. mayonnaise
- 2 oz. sour cream
- Seasoning:
- 1/3 tsp salt
- ¼ tsp ground black pepper
- ¼ tsp hot sauce

Directions:

1. Take a medium bowl, place cream cheese in it, add mayonnaise, sour cream, salt, black pepper and hot sauce and stir until well combined.
2. Add zucchini noodles, toss until well coated and then fold in salmon until just mixed.
3. Serve.

Nutrition: 458 Calories; 38.7 g Fats; 15.4 g Protein; 6.1 g Net Carb; 1.7 g Fiber;

25. Tuna Salad Pickle Boats

Preparation Time: 10 minutes

Cooking Time: 0 minutes;

Servings: 2

Ingredients

- 4 dill pickles
- 4 oz. of tuna, packed in water, drained
- ¼ of lime, juiced
- 4 tbsp. mayonnaise
- Seasoning:
- ¼ tsp salt
- 1/8 tsp ground black pepper
- ¼ tsp paprika
- 1 tbsp. mustard paste

Directions:

1. Prepare tuna salad and for this, take a medium bowl, place tuna in it, add lime juice, mayonnaise, salt, black pepper, paprika, and mustard and stir until mixed.
2. Cut each pickle into half lengthwise, scoop out seeds, and then fill with tuna salad.

3. Serve.

Nutrition: 308.5 Calories; 23.7 g Fats; 17 g Protein; 3.8 g Net Carb; 3.1 g Fiber;

26. Shrimp Deviled Eggs

Preparation Time: 5 minutes

Cooking Time: 0 minutes;

Servings: 2

Ingredients

- 2 eggs, boiled
- 2 oz. shrimps, cooked, chopped
- ½ tsp tabasco sauce
- ½ tsp mustard paste
- 2 tbsp. mayonnaise
- Seasoning:
- 1/8 tsp salt
- 1/8 tsp ground black pepper

Directions:

1. Peel the boiled eggs, then slice in half lengthwise and transfer egg yolks to a medium bowl by using a spoon.
2. Mash the egg yolk, add remaining ingredients and stir until well combined.
3. Spoon the egg yolk mixture into egg whites, and then serve.

Nutrition: 210 Calories; 16.4 g Fats; 14 g Protein; 1 g Net Carb; 0.1 g Fiber;

27. Herb Crusted Tilapia

Preparation Time: 5 minutes

Cooking Time: 10 minutes;

Servings: 2

Ingredients

- 2 fillets of tilapia
- ½ tsp garlic powder
- ½ tsp Italian seasoning
- ½ tsp dried parsley
- 1/3 tsp salt
- Seasoning:
- 2 tbsp. melted butter, unsalted
- 1 tbsp. avocado oil

Directions:

1. Turn on the broiler and then let it preheat.
2. Meanwhile, take a small bowl, place melted butter in it, stir in oil and garlic powder until mixed, and then brush this mixture over tilapia fillets.
3. Stir together remaining spices and then sprinkle them generously on tilapia until well coated.

4. Place seasoned tilapia in a baking pan, place the pan under the broiler and then bake for 10 minutes until tender and golden, brushing with garlic-butter every 2 minutes.
5. Serve.

Nutrition: 520 Calories; 35 g Fats; 36.2 g Protein; 13.6 g Net Carb; 0.6 g Fiber;

28. Tuna Stuffed Avocado

Preparation Time: 5 minutes

Cooking Time: 0 minutes;

Servings: 2

Ingredients

- 1 medium avocado
- ¼ of a lemon, juiced
- 5-ounce tuna, packed in water
- 1 green onion, chopped
- 2 slices of turkey bacon, cooked, crumbled
- Seasoning:
- ¼ tsp salt
- ¼ tsp ground black pepper

Directions:

1. Drain tuna, place it in a bowl, and then broke it into pieces with a form.
2. Add remaining ingredients, except for avocado and bacon, and stir until well combined.
3. Cut avocado into half, remove its pit and then stuff its cavity evenly with the tuna mixture.
4. Top stuffed avocados with bacon and Serve.

Nutrition: 108.5 Calories; 8 g Fats; 6 g Protein; 0.8 g Net Carb; 2.3 g Fiber;

VEGETABLES

29. Garlicky Green Beans

Preparation Time: 10 minutes

Cooking Time: 10 minutes

Servings: 4

Ingredients:

- 1 pound green beans, stemmed
- 2 tablespoons olive oil
- 1 teaspoon minced garlic
- Sea salt
- Freshly ground black pepper
- ¼ cup freshly grated Parmesan cheese

Directions:

1. Preheat the oven to 425°F. Line a baking sheet with aluminum foil and set aside.
2. In a large bowl, toss together the green beans, olive oil, and garlic until well mixed.
3. Season the beans lightly with salt and pepper

4. Spread the beans on the baking sheet and roast them until they are tender and lightly browned, stirring them once, about 10 minutes.
5. Serve topped with the Parmesan cheese.

Nutrition: Calories: 104 Fat: 9g Protein: 4g Carbs: 2g Fiber: 1g Net Carbs: 1g Fat 77 Protein 15 Carbs 8

30. Sautéed Asparagus with Walnuts

Preparation Time: 10 minutes

Cooking Time: 5 minutes

Servings: 4

Ingredients:

- 1½ tablespoons olive oil
- ¾ pound asparagus, woody ends trimmed
- Sea salt
- Freshly ground pepper
- ¼ cup chopped walnuts

Directions:

1. Place a large skillet over medium-high heat and add the olive oil.
2. Sauté the asparagus until the spears are tender and lightly browned, about 5 minutes.
3. Season the asparagus with salt and pepper.
4. Remove the skillet from the heat and toss the asparagus with the walnuts.
5. Serve.

Nutrition: Calories: 124 Fat: 12g Protein: 3g Carbs: 4g Fiber: 2g Net Carbs: 2g Fat 81 Protein Carbs 10

31. Brussels Sprouts Casserole

Preparation Time: 15 minutes

Cooking Time: 30 minutes

Servings: 8

Ingredients:

- 8 bacon slices
- 1 pound Brussels sprouts, blanched for 10 minutes and cut into quarters
- 1 cup shredded Swiss cheese, divided
- ¾ cup heavy (whipping) cream

Directions:

1. Preheat the oven to 400°F.
2. Place a skillet over medium-high heat and cook the bacon until it is crispy, about 6 minutes.
3. Reserve 1 tablespoon of bacon fat to grease the casserole dish and roughly chop the cooked bacon.
4. Lightly oil a casserole dish with the reserved bacon fat and set aside.

5. In a medium bowl, toss the Brussels sprouts with the chopped bacon and ½ cup of cheese and transfer the mixture to the casserole dish.
6. Pour the heavy cream over the Brussels sprouts and top the casserole with the remaining ½ cup of cheese.
7. Bake until the cheese is melted and lightly browned and the vegetables are heated through, about 20 minutes.
8. Serve.

Nutrition: Calories: 299 Fat: 11g Protein: 12g Carbs: 7gFiber: 3g Net Carbs: 4g Fat 77 Protein 15 Carbs 8

32. Cheesy Mashed Cauliflower

Preparation Time: 15 minutes

Cooking Time: 5 minutes

Servings: 4

Ingredients:

- 1 head cauliflower, chopped roughly
- ½ cup shredded Cheddar cheese
- ¼ cup heavy (whipping) cream
- 2 tablespoons butter, at room temperature
- Sea salt
- Freshly ground black pepper

Directions:

1. Place a large saucepan filled three-quarters full with water over high heat and bring to a boil.
2. Blanch the cauliflower until tender, about 5 minutes, and drain.
3. Transfer the cauliflower to a food processor and add the cheese, heavy cream, and butter. Purée until very creamy and whipped.
4. Season with salt and pepper.
5. Serve.

Nutrition: Calories: 183 Fat: 15g Protein: 8g Carbs: 6g Fiber: 2g Net Carbs: 4g Fat 75 Protein 14 Carbs 11

33. Egg Broth

Preparation Time: 5 minutes

Cooking Time: 5 minutes

Servings: 4

Ingredients:

- 2 tablespoons unsalted butter
- 4 cups chicken broth
- 3 large eggs
- Salt and black pepper, to taste
- 1 sliced green onion, for garnish

Directions:

1. Take a medium stockpot and place it over high heat.
2. Add butter and chicken broth to the pot and bring to a boil.
3. Break eggs into a bowl and beat them for 1 minute with a fork until frothy.
4. Once the broth boils, slowly pour in beaten eggs while stirring the broth with a spoon.
5. Cook for 1 minute with continuously stirring, then sprinkle salt and black pepper to season.

6. Garnish with sliced green onion, then serve warm.

Nutrition: Calories: 93 Fat: 7.8g Total carbs: 1.8g Fiber: 0.1g Protein: 3.9g

34. Cauliflower Cream Soup

Preparation Time: 15 minutes

Cooking Time: 4 hours 10 minutes

Servings: 5

Ingredients:

- 10 slices bacon
- 3 small heads cauliflower, cored and cut into florets
- 4 cups chicken broth
- ¼ cup (½ stick) salted butter
- 3 cloves garlic, pressed
- ½ large yellow onion, chopped
- 1 cup heavy whipping cream
- 2 cups Cheddar cheese, shredded
- Salt and black pepper, to taste
- Freshly chopped chives or green onions, for garnish

Directions:

1. Take a large skillet and place it over medium heat.

2. Add bacon to the skillet and cook for about 8 minutes until brown and crispy.
3. Transfer the cooked bacon to a paper towel-lined plate to absorb the excess grease.
4. Allow the bacon to cool, then chop it. Wrap the plate of chopped bacon in plastic and refrigerate it.
5. Add the cauliflower florets to the food processor and pulse until chopped thoroughly.
6. Add chicken broth, butter, garlic, onion, and chopped cauliflower to the slow cooker.
7. Give all these ingredients a gentle stir, then put on the lid.
8. Cook the cauliflower soup for 4 hours on high heat.
9. Once the cauliflower is tender, purée the soup with an immersion blender until smooth.
10. Add chopped bacon, heavy cream, cheese, salt, and black pepper. Mix well and let the cheese melt in the hot soup.
11. Garnish with green onions or chives, then serve warm.

Nutrition: Calories: 627 Fat: 54.3g Total carbs: 13.7gFiber: 3.7g

Protein: 24.6g

35. Shrimp Mushroom Chowder

Preparation Time: 10 minutes

Cooking Time: 40 minutes

Servings: 6

Ingredients:

- ¼ cup refined avocado oil
- 1/3 cup diced yellow onions
- 1 2/3 cups diced mushrooms
- 10½ ounces (298 g) small raw shrimp, shelled and deveined
- 1 can (131/2-ounce / 383-g) unsweetened coconut milk
- 1/3 cup chicken bone broth
- 2 tablespoons apple cider vinegar
- 1 teaspoon onion powder
- 1 teaspoon paprika
- 1 bay leaf
- ¾ teaspoon finely ground gray sea salt
- ½ teaspoon dried oregano leaves
- ¼ teaspoon ground black pepper
- 1 medium zucchini (7-ounce / 198-g), cubed
- 12 radishes (6-ounce / 170-g), cubed

Directions:

1. Add avocado oil to a large saucepan and place it over medium heat.
2. Add onions and mushrooms to the pan and sauté for 10 minutes or until onions are soft and mushrooms are lightly browned.
3. Stir in shrimp, coconut milk, chicken broth, apple cider vinegar, onion powder, paprika, bay leaf, sea salt, oregano leaves, and black pepper.
4. Cover the soup mixture with a lid and cook for 20 minutes on low heat.
5. Add zucchini and radishes to the soup and cook for 10 minutes.
6. Remove the bay leaf from the soup and divide the soup into 6 small serving bowls. Serve hot.

Nutrition: Calories: 311 Fat: 26.3g Total carbs: 7.7g Fiber: 2.9g Protein: 13.7g

36. Pork Tarragon Soup

Preparation Time: 10 minutes

Cooking Time: 1 hour 20 minutes

Servings: 6

Ingredients:

- 1/3 cup lard
- 1 pound (454 g) pork loin, cut into ½-inch (1.25-cm) pieces
- 10 strips bacon (about 10-ounce / 284-g), cut into ½-inch (1.25-cm) pieces
- ¾ cup sliced shallots
- 3 medium turnips (about 12½-ounce / 354-g), cubed
- 1 tablespoon yellow mustard
- ¼ cup dry white wine
- 1¾ cups chicken bone broth
- 4 sprigs fresh thyme
- 2 tablespoons unflavored gelatin
- 2 tablespoons apple cider vinegar
- ½ cup unsweetened coconut milk
- 1 tablespoon dried tarragon leaves

Directions:

1. Take a large saucepan and place it over medium heat.
2. Add lard to the saucepan and allow it to melt.
3. Add pork pieces to the melted lard and sauté for 8 minutes until golden brown.
4. Add bacon pieces and sliced shallots and sauté for 5 minutes or until fragrant.
5. Add turnips, mustard, wine, bone broth, and thyme sprigs to the soup.
6. Mix these ingredients gently and cover this soup with a lid.
7. Bring the soup to a boil, then reduce the heat to medium-low. Cook this soup for 1 hour.
8. Remove and discard the thyme sprigs from the soup then add gelatin, vinegar, coconut milk, and tarragon.
9. Increase the heat to medium and bring the soup to a boil. Cover to cook for 10 minutes.
10. Divide the cooked soup into 6 serving bowls and serve warm.

Nutrition: Calories: 566 Fat: 41.5g Total carbs: 9.7gFiber: 1.2g Protein: 39.6g

37. Creamy Broccoli and Cauliflower Soup

Preparation Time: 20 minutes

Cooking Time: 15 minutes

Servings: 6

Ingredients:

- 1 (13½-ounce / 383-g) can unsweetened coconut milk
- 2 cups vegetable stock
- 1 (14-ounce / 397-g) small head cauliflower, cored and cut into large florets
- 2 medium celery sticks, chopped
- 1 teaspoon finely ground gray sea salt
- 6 green onions, green parts only, roughly chopped
- 1 large head broccoli, cored and cut into large florets
- ¼ teaspoon ground black pepper
- ¼ teaspoon ground white pepper
- 1/3 cup butter-infused olive oil
- 1 chopped green onion, for garnish

Directions:

1. Take a large saucepan and place it over medium heat.
2. Add coconut milk, vegetable stock, cauliflower florets, chopped celery, salt, and green onions.
3. Mix them gently, then cover and bring the soup to a boil.
4. Continue cooking the soup for 15 minutes until the cauliflower florets are soft.
5. Meanwhile, blanch the broccoli in a pot of boiling water for 1 minute until soft but still crisp, then drain on a paper towel. Set aside on a plate.
6. When the cauliflower soup is cooked, transfer it to a blender.
7. Add black pepper, white pepper, and olive oil. Blend the soup for 1 minute until smooth.
8. Add the soft broccoli and blend again for 30 seconds.
9. Divide the cooked broccoli and cauliflower soup into 6 serving bowls.
10. Garnish with chopped green onions and serve warm.

Nutrition: Calories: 264 Fat: 23.3g Total carbs: 10.3g Fiber: 3.6g Protein: 6.9g

38. Chicken Turnip Soup

Preparation Time: 10 minutes

Cooking Time: 6 to 8 hours

Servings: 5

Ingredients:

- 12 ounces (340g) bone-in chicken
- ¼ cup turnip, chopped
- ¼ cup onions, chopped
- 4 garlic cloves, smashed
- 4 cups water
- 3 sprigs thyme
- 2 bay leaves
- Salt, to taste
- ¼ teaspoon freshly ground black pepper

Directions:

1. Put the chicken, turnip, onions, garlic, water, thyme springs, and bay leaves in a slow cooker.
2. Season with salt and pepper, then give the mixture a good stir.
3. Cover and cook on low for 6 to 8 hours until the chicken is cooked through.

4. When ready, remove the bay leaves and shred the chicken with a fork.
5. Divide the soup among five bowls and serve.

Nutrition: Calories: 186 Fat: 13.6g Total carbs: 3.3g Fiber: 2.6g Protein: 15.2g

39. Spinach Mushroom Soup

Preparation Time: 10 minutes

Cooking Time: 5 minutes

Servings: 3

Ingredients:

- 1 tablespoon olive oil
- 1 teaspoon garlic, finely chopped
- 1 cup spinach, torn into small pieces
- ½ cup mushrooms, chopped
- Salt and freshly ground black pepper, to taste
- ½ teaspoon tamari
- 3 cups vegetable stock
- 1 teaspoon sesame seeds, roasted

Directions:

1. Place a saucepan over medium heat and add olive oil to heat.
2. Add garlic to the hot oil and sauté for 30 seconds or until fragrant.
3. Add spinach and mushrooms, then sauté for 1 minute or until lightly tender.

4. Add salt, black pepper, tamari, and vegetable stock. Cook for another 3 minutes. Stir constantly.
5. Garnish with sesame seeds and serve warm.

Nutrition: Calories: 80 Fat: 7.4g Total carbs: 3.2g Fiber: 1.1g Protein: 1.2g

40. Garlicky Chicken Soup

Preparation Time: 10 minutes

Cooking Time: 10 minutes

Servings: 4

Ingredients:

- 2 tablespoons butter
- 1 large chicken breast cut into strips
- 4 ounces (113 g) cream cheese, cubed
- 2 tablespoons Garlic Gusto Seasoning
- ½ cup heavy cream
- 14½ ounces (411 g) chicken broth
- Salt, to taste

Directions:

1. Place a saucepan over medium heat and add butter to melt.
2. Add chicken strips and sauté for 2 minutes.
3. Add cream cheese and seasoning, and cook for 3 minutes, stirring occasionally.
4. Pour in the heavy cream and chicken broth. Bring the soup to a boil, then lower the heat.

5. Allow the soup to simmer for 4 minutes, then sprinkle with salt.
6. Let cool for 5 minutes and serve while warm.

Nutrition: Calories: 243 Fat: 22.5g Total carbs: 7.0gFiber: 6.6g Protein: 9.6g

DESSERTS

41. Vanilla Almond Ice Pops

Preparation Time: 10 minutes + 4 hours chilling

Cooking Time: 15 minutes

Servings: 18

Ingredients:

- 2 cups almond milk
- 1 cup heavy (whipping) cream
- 1 vanilla bean, halved lengthwise
- 1 cup shredded unsweetened coconut

Directions:

1. Set a medium saucepan on medium heat, then put the almond milk, heavy cream, and vanilla bean.
2. Bring the liquid to a simmer and reduce the heat to low. Continue to simmer for 5 minutes.
3. Remove the saucepan from the heat and let the liquid cool.

4. Take the vanilla bean out of the liquid and use a knife to scrape the seeds out of the bean into the liquid.
5. Stir in the coconut and divide the liquid between the ice pop molds.
6. Freeze until solid, about 4 hours, and enjoy.

Nutrition: Calories: 166 Fat: 15g Protein: 3g Carbs: 4g Fiber: 2g Net Carbs: 2g

42. Peanut Butter Fudge Cake

Preparation Time: 10 minutes + 3 hours chilling

Cooking Time: 0 minutes

Servings: 8

Ingredients:

- 3/4 cup peanut butter, sugar-free, preferably homemade
- 3 tablespoons cocoa nibs, unsweetened and melted
- 1/4 teaspoon baking powder
- 3 tablespoons coconut oil, at room temperature
- 1 teaspoon vanilla extract
- 1 stick butter
- 1/3 cup almond milk
- 1/3 cup Swerve
- A pinch of salt
- A pinch of grated nutmeg

Directions:

1. Melt the butter in your microwave. Stir in the milk, 1/4 cup of Swerve, salt, nutmeg, and baking powder.

2. Spoon the batter into a parchment-lined baking dish. Refrigerate for about 3 hours or until set.
3. Meanwhile, make the sauce by whisking the remaining ingredients until everything is well incorporated.
4. Spoon the sauce over your fudge cake.

Nutrition: 180 Calories 18.3g Fat 4.5g Carbs 1g Protein 1.1g Fiber

43. Rum Chocolate Pralines

Preparation Time: 10 minutes + chilling time

Cooking Time: 0 minutes

Servings: 8

Ingredients:

- 1 cup bakers' chocolate, sugar-free
- 2 tablespoons dark rum
- 1/8 teaspoon ground cloves
- 1/8 teaspoon cinnamon powder
- 1/2 teaspoon almond extract
- 1/2 teaspoon rum extract
- 2 tablespoons cocoa powder
- 1/4 cup almond butter
- 1 cup almond milk

Directions:

1. Microwave the chocolate, cocoa, and almond butter until they have completely melted.
2. Add in the other ingredients and mix to combine well. Pour the mixture into silicone molds and place them in your refrigerator until set.

Nutrition: 70 Calories 3.4g Fat 5.1g Carbs 2.4g Protein 1.6g Fiber

SMOOTHIES AND DRINKS

44. Strawberry zucchini chia smoothie

Preparation Time: 11 minutes

Cooking Time: 0 minutes

Servings: 1

Ingredients:

- 1 cup of water
- 1/2 cup of frozen strawberries
- 1 cup of chopped zucchini, frozen or raw
- 1 tbsp. of chia seeds

Directions:

1. To a high-speed blender, add all the smoothie ingredients and blend until smooth and combined.
2. Serve immediately and enjoy!

Nutrition: 19 calories 9g fat 9g carbohydrates 7g protein

45. Chocolate Peanut Butter Smoothie

Preparation Time: 5 minutes

Cooking Time: 0 minutes

Servings: 3

Ingredients:

- 1/4 cup peanut butter (creamy)
- 3 tbsp. cocoa powder
- 1 cup heavy cream
- 1 1/2 cup unsweetened almond milk
- 6 tbsp. sweetener or to taste
- 1/8 tsp sea salt (optional)

Directions:

1. To a high-speed blender, add all the smoothie ingredients and blend until smooth and combined.
2. Serve immediately and enjoy!

Nutrition: 435 calories 41g fat 6g carbohydrates 9g protein

46. Blueberry Coconut Chia Smoothies

Preparation Time: 11 minutes

Cooking Time: 0 minutes

Servings: 4

Ingredients:

- 1 cup frozen blueberries
- 1 cup full-fat Greek yogurt
- 1/2 cup coconut cream
- 1 cup unsweetened cashew or almond milk
- 2 tbsp. coconut oil
- 2 tbsp. ground chia seed
- 2 tbsp. swerve sweetener

Directions:

1. To a high-speed blender, add all the smoothie ingredients and blend until smooth and combined.
2. Serve immediately and enjoy!

Nutrition: 249 calories 21.07g fat 11.26g carbohydrates 6.23g protein

47. Coconut Milk Strawberry Smoothie

Preparation Time: 2 minutes

Cooking Time: 0 minutes

Servings: 2

Ingredients:

- 1 cup strawberries frozen
- 1 cup unsweetened coconut milk
- 2 tbsp. smooth almond butter
- 2 packets stevia optional

Directions:

1. Place all together the ingredients into the food processor and blend until pureed.

Nutrition: 397 calories 37g fat 15g carbohydrates 6g protein

48. Vanilla Intermittent Smoothie

Preparation Time: 11 minutes

Cooking Time: 0 minutes

Servings: 1

Ingredients:

- 1 13.5-oz (400ml) can coconut milk
- 1 cup heavy cream
- 1/4 cup sweetener or to taste
- 2 tsp vanilla extract
- 2 cups ice cubes

Directions:

1. Put all together the ingredients in a blender and blend until pureed.

Nutrition: 379 calories 38g fat 4g carbohydrates 3g protein

49. Raspberry Protein Shake (soy)

Preparation Time: 5 minutes

Cooking Time: 0 minutes

Servings: 1

Ingredients:

- 1 cup full-fat coconut milk (or alternatively, use almond milk)
- Optional: ¼ cup coconut cream
- 1 scoop organic soy protein (chocolate or vanilla flavor)
- ½ cup raspberries (fresh or frozen)
- 1 tbsp. low-carb maple syrup
- Optional: 2-4 ice cubes

Directions:

1. Add all the ingredients to a blender, including the optional coconut cream and ice cubes if desired, and blend for 1 minute.
2. Transfer the shake to a large cup or shaker, and enjoy!
3. Alternatively, store the smoothie in an airtight container or a mason jar, keep it in the fridge, and consume within 2 days. Store for a

maximum of 30 days in the freezer and thaw at room temperature.

Nutrition: Calories: 311 kcal Net Carbs: 6.9 g. Fat: 19.3 g. Protein: 26.8 g. Fiber: 5 g. Sugar: 4.8 g.

50. Forest Fruit Blaster (soy)

Preparation Time: 5 minutes

Cooking Time: 0 minutes

Servings: 1

Ingredients:

- ¼ cup mixed berries (fresh or frozen)
- ½ kiwi (peeled)
- 2 cups full-fat coconut milk
- 2 scoops organic soy protein (vanilla flavor)
- ½ cup water
- Optional: 2 ice cubes

Directions:

1. Add all the ingredients to a blender, including the optional ice if desired, and blend for 1 minute.
2. Transfer the shake to a large cup or shaker and enjoy!
3. Alternatively, store the smoothie in an airtight container or a mason jar, keep it in the fridge, and consume within 2 days. Store for a maximum of 30 days in the freezer and thaw at room temperature.

Nutrition: Calories: 603 kcal Net Carbs: 11.5 g. Fat: 38.1 g. Protein: 52.9 g. Fiber: 4.5 g. Sugar: 9.9 g.

CPSIA information can be obtained
at www.ICGtesting.com
Printed in the USA
LVHW020959290521
688874LV00028B/1729

9 781801 839914